HEALING FROM ACID REFLUX

JOANNA SANDERS

Cover Design, Editing, Formatting: Joanna Sanders, LLC www.colossians46.com

All true credit and glory to Jesus the Healer.

ISBN (Paperback): 978-1-7342932-6-5

ISBN (eBook): 978-1-7342932-8-9

HEALING FROM ACID REFLUX

JOANNA SANDERS

To Jesus, my Healer

✝

To my dad, in celebration of your ultimate healing,

✝

To my husband, for being the daily manifestation of His love.

Joanna

HEALING FROM ACID REFLUX

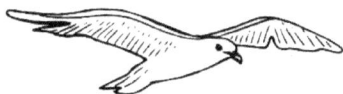

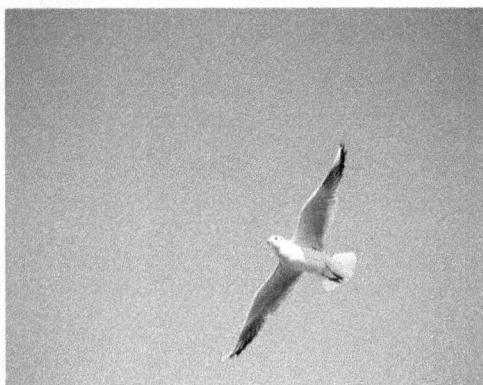

Introduction

This is meant to be a short read for you. I want to keep it simple, because it's likely you're looking for answers, and have already spent time looking elsewhere. Your time is precious. I'm going to present the answer you're looking for, right up front, and then I'm going to walk you through my experience with that answer.

The answer for your healing is in Jesus Christ alone. You do not have to agree with that for it to still be true. I know it to be true and I hope you hear through my experience why I'm so certain.

Mine has not been a miraculous overnight healing. That's not to say that yours won't be, as all things are possible with Him (Matt 19:26). But for me, it's been a step-by-step journey as I learned to abide with Him, through this "condition." The journey on my own, prior to that, had been one of fear and of death. When I started walking through it with Him, it became such a small aspect of my life that I truly didn't even consider it a problem anymore; I considered it a victory. That major transition is what I want to share with you—because no matter what anyone has told you about your condition, (and truly whatever your condition is), walking through it with Jesus Christ will turn the darkness to light.

My journey with acid reflux now, is light. Nothing else. He's taken the heavy burden as He promised and given me the light one. (See Matthew 11:28-30.) Even if someday, I die of this very condition, the burden is light.

So, the most important aspect of the book has already been covered: Jesus is the Healer. Next, I will explain the process He took me through to the victory and the incredible freedom in my healing.

The first chapter will be my family history, because I had reason to be scared based on my bloodline. The threat of complications with me was real. Next, I'm going to walk you through my medicinal management of it and the side effects I experienced along the way. After that, I'm going to explain how I knew to come off my prescription medications, and the exact process I used to do it. I'll also explain the lifestyle changes I made to support my healing and what it all looks like now from the other side, including what over-the-counter medications I take, and how I manage it with diet, supplements, prayer, and mindset.

Before you read on, I must emphasize the "disclaimer" part of this book. This is in no way medical advice for you. I am not a doctor, and I am no longer a certified personal fitness trainer. I am not medically qualified to give advice. This is my story, and mine alone. In terms of medical results, I am not implying in any way that following my path will give you the same results, or will even be safe for you. Ultimately, that's between you and God, and any qualified physician that He's assigned to tend to you. Spiritually though, I can guarantee that walking this out with Christ will show you the path to victory and freedom, even if at the end of the day, you still have reflux. I can guarantee that because I am an ambassador for Christ, and He promises all of that and more, in His Word.

So if the Son sets you free, you will be free indeed.

John 8:36

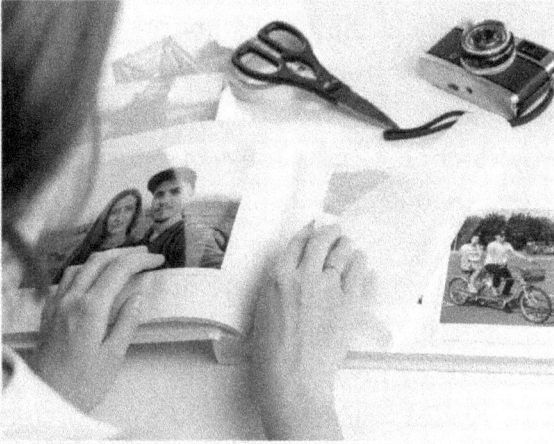

Family History

I was twenty-four years old when my father died of esophageal cancer. He was fifty-six, and the loss was quick and devastating. Several years prior, my great uncle—who was his first uncle, died of the same thing. My mother had dealt with reflux and regular throat-clearing for as long as I could remember. So, when I started showing heartburn symptoms in my early twenties, the doctors were cautious and aggressive.

They did an endoscopy on me, which showed inflammation but was otherwise clear. They put me on prescription proton pump inhibitors and told me I would be on these the rest of my life. They told me this was the better alternative to the implied path my dad experienced. They also told me that I would need endoscopies done every couple of years or so for the rest of my life to keep watch.

In my background, there are two other things that should also be considered. First, is my ethnic heritage. Both of my parents were Italian, so I grew up with a typical Italian diet of red tomato sauce, red wine, sometimes greasy foods, and oils. While my mom did the best she could to teach us good eating habits, I loved eating late at night (when I was always most hungry), I didn't drink a lot of water, and when I was in my late teens and twenties, I would drink alcohol with my friends three to four nights a week, and then go out to eat after the club closed at 2:00 or 3:00am. Occasionally, I also smoked. A perfect storm, these were all really bad habits for someone with a history of this type of cancer. But being young and naïve, I believed that as long as I took the daily medication they had prescribed for me, I was free and clear. I should also mention that these unhealthy habits were all before I submitted my heart and my life to Christ. (Now I understand what proper stewardship looks like from His perspective, as my body is no longer my own.)

The second factor is that my dad worked in a nuclear facility for some time when I was young. I don't remember what work my uncle did. Some doctors speculated that exposure at that facility could have led to the growth of the deadly tumor in my dad's esophagus. My dad was a social drinker, and later in his life also had the occasional cigarette or cigar. He was within a healthy weight range, was active, and all other aspects of his physical health were good, including bloodwork just a few months prior to the discovery of the tumor. His diagnosis was completely unexpected, and even though they were optimistic at the beginning of his treatment, especially after his surgery, it was only six months from the time of his diagnosis to the time of his death. Every single thing they believed would help ended up being disastrous. It was a horrific downward spiral of hopeful claims and tragic results.

I now am at peace with his death—something I'd never thought I'd say. It's been twenty years since he died, and I remember thinking that I wouldn't survive a day without him. God has given me complete peace about it, which is also something only He could have done.

In hindsight, several other family members seemed to also suffer from heartburn symptoms, and reflux in general. It was so common in my family that it didn't seem to alarm anyone until my dad died.

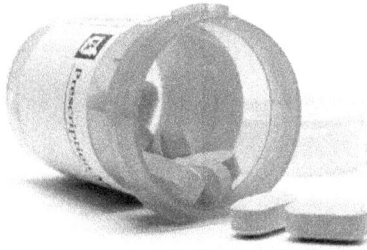

Medicinal Management

After showing symptoms for acid reflux in my mid-twenties, around the time that my dad died, I was put on daily prescription meds that I was told I would have to take for the rest of my life. I knew absolutely nothing about these proton pump inhibitors except that they came with a clearly implied promise that I could eat whatever I want and not have to worry about getting cancer like my dad did. My journey with prescription proton pump inhibitors lasted twenty years.

After twenty years on prescription proton pump inhibitors, I experienced almost every long-term side effect that is documented, and each of the meds lost efficacy for me after a year or two. I literally tried every medication on the market, and would have to shuffle through the list again, or change combinations of them after they became ineffective once more.

While I encourage you to research the long-term side effects of these types of medications, I can share what I experienced. Again, I am not claiming to be providing any sort of medical advice, nor am I claiming that these were all related to my long-term use of proton-pump inhibitors. This was just my experience.

During the two decades of taking these meds, I became anemic and had to take iron supplements regularly. I also developed a severe list of allergies to foods and other medications. At one point, my allergies got so bad that I literally became allergic to my own sweat and would break out in massive hives almost daily. (Not a joke. I did seek treatment from an allergy doctor after that and have since been healed from that too.) I had difficulty sleeping from time to time and was often tired a lot. I had to have major dental work in these two decades due to weak or "soft enamel." I was borderline for high-blood pressure. During these two decades, my eyesight also got progressively worse, which I chalked up to aging.

In the last few years of these meds, I would occasionally have "flare-ups" where my reflux would get so bad that I would have a hoarse throat and voice and dry coughing regularly throughout the day, including at night while I was trying to sleep. The hoarse voice became embarrassing in public or over the phone, as it was difficult to talk clearly. This would happen a couple times a year and sometimes last two to three months.

When the flare-ups would occur, or the medication I was currently on began to prove ineffective, I would be told to double up on the meds, or add in additional ones, or add in over-the-counter medications as well. At my worst, I was on two daily prescription medications as well as over-the-counter meds to supplement. The overall pattern was that the longer I was on these prescription medications the more difficult things became to manage, and the more side effects I was having.

During this time (the twenty years I took the proton pump inhibitors), I did not alter my eating habits much. I still drank alcohol two-to-three times per week. I was a regular and religious coffee drinker (two to four cups per day). At one point, I worked managing a winery, and the job right after that was selling chocolate; so I was clearly not avoiding any trigger foods, and had even made a lifestyle around them. I still ate heavy meals at times and ate late at night when I had the opportunity. I ate what I wanted and when I wanted. I smoked only very occasionally.

I worked out on a regular basis most of this time, and I had an active lifestyle. My weight was stable and within a generally healthy range for my height, so it wasn't a drastic change in diet or weight gain that was significantly impacting any of these symptoms. However, I will note that when I was at the higher end of my weight range and my clothes were tighter, my symptoms were usually more pronounced.

One could easily argue that my lifestyle was not supportive of my condition improving, and that was why things got worse, not better. One could easily argue that the medication was not the problem, but rather my own lifestyle choices. That would be a legitimate argument, even though it doesn't account for the many other health effects that were noted. However, for me, that position just reaffirms the saving grace of Jesus Christ to heal me despite me. If I had not experienced such a massive change in health once I submitted my body to Him and allowed Him to show me how to steward it properly, I would not be claiming my healing today.

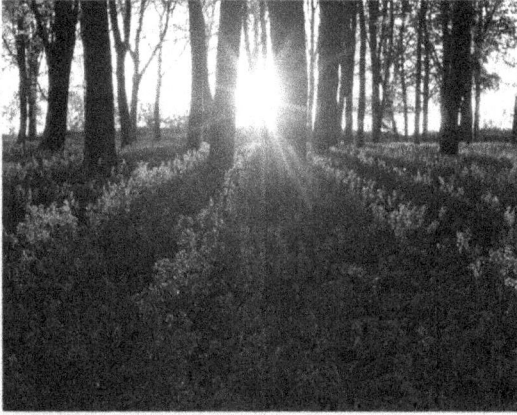

Revelation

It wasn't until well after I got saved and submitted my life to Christ, that I started to question whether or not the long-term use of the prescription meds were really the best stewardship over my body. As a believer in Christ, I submit to the Scripture in 1 Corinthians 6:19-20, which states:

Do you not know that your bodies are temples of the Holy Spirit, who is in you, whom you have received from God? You are not your own; you were bought at a price. Therefore honor God with your bodies.

I began to reflect and realized that honoring God with my body meant that I submitted to God first, and not man. Even though I believed that I had trustworthy and well-intended doctors, I had never really asked God if this was the path He had wanted me to take for treatment. And after experiencing many side effects, I eventually had to admit that this couldn't have been good stewardship, especially when I knew there were other lifestyle choices I could make that would help drastically. I wasn't sure at the time that my problems would be entirely eliminated by lifestyle changes, but I was sensing that the current medicinal path was no longer effective on its own.

Spiritually, I knew something was breaking through. Physically, I was tired of the flare-ups which did not seem under control, and I was especially alarmed when the next level of prescription options was a cholesterol medication with the side effect of lowering acid production in the body. (My cholesterol was fine.) I knew that medication would also come with a whole other host of side effects and sooner than later I'd need more medication to manage them. Something wasn't sitting right anymore. I began to research and it was in my research that I realized my problem wasn't actually acid; it was reflux. And those are separate issues, but they are typically grouped together because of the way they interact in digestion.

The breakthrough came during a flare-up which lasted more than three months. I had developed a regular intermittent dry cough that was disruptive to my daily activities and prohibited me from sleeping well at night. I had no heartburn symptoms, and my digestion seemed fine. I didn't have cold symptoms other than the seasonal allergies I had been used to dealing with. Even so, I tried every cough and cold medication on the market. I saw various specialists. I was tested for asthma and put on an inhaler. I switched up my proton pump inhibitor once more just in case. I finally made a follow-up appointment with my allergist, and she happened to ask me if I had reflux. I was surprised by the question because I had never heard of a dry cough being related to reflux, but I was glad she asked. I told her of my long-term use of proton pump inhibitors, and she suggested I try Gaviscon, which is an over-the-counter medication. Within days, my horrible cough was gone. I was floored, and I started to research how, and why, the Gaviscon worked when nothing else would.

In my research, I found that the Gaviscon operated differently than the proton pump inhibitors. The Gaviscon would actually form a barrier over the contents of my stomach to stop them from refluxing. It wasn't focused on the acid, as my prescription medications had been. It was focused on the reflux. (Please note there are several versions of Gaviscon available, and it's important to understand the differences. I will cover the specifics in the next chapter.)

I then recalled that one endoscopy that I had showed that I had a weak LES sphincter. In layman's terms, that means that the valve (it's actually a muscle) that keeps the stomach contents down wasn't a very strong lid in my case. So even when I didn't eat much, or ate all the right things, the valve that was supposed to keep everything down in my stomach, wasn't necessarily closing all the way, and reflux was happening one way or another. The Gaviscon worked because it basically did what my LES sphincter was supposed to do.

I went into serious research mode, and I learned a lot. I'm sharing what I learned here in the hopes that this may help someone as it helped me, but I am not claiming to have any medical qualifications for this information. I can't even claim that I'm certain it is all completely accurate as I took from many sources to gain this knowledge. Please do your own research and verify with a trusted and qualified physician before making any changes in your own life. And I believe it is most important to pray.

I learned that Laryngopharyngeal Reflux, or LPR for short, was basically reflux that went way past the stomach and lower esophagus area, and could extend to the voice box, and even into the sinuses and the dental area. It could cause coughing, a hoarse voice, and even extensive sinus and allergy symptoms. It could also cause dental problems! LPR rarely produces heartburn-like symptoms, which is why another name for it is "silent reflux." And it can be just as dangerous as chronic acid-reflux heartburn symptoms. From my research, I learned that you can block acid as much as you want (even though your body is going to still produce it because it needs it to digest), yet if you are refluxing, you still have a problem on your hands, because it's not just acid that causes issues when it doesn't stay in the stomach, it's also pepsin.

Pepsin is a major digestive enzyme that is critical to digestion, especially with proteins. The combination of acid and pepsin is what helps to digest our food properly. LPR happens when the pressure in the stomach outweighs the tone (strength) of the LES, and therefore refluxing occurs. If your acid content is low, then when you reflux, the acid won't be as much of a concern. But even if the acid is low, pepsin is still present, and pepsin outside of the digestive system can be equally problematic. Now, there is a bit more to this, especially in understanding how the pepsin needs an acidic environment to thrive—but for the purpose of this short book I won't go into all those details. Please research more on your own if you are curious.

My conclusion was that the medication I had taken for twenty years was only targeting one side effect of the actual problem. My actual problem was reflux (in my case, mainly LPR) and the combination of both pepsin and acid in areas where they shouldn't be was causing all sorts of issues in various places in my body. This was the revelation for me that I needed to target the reflux—and not just the acid. In fact, this revelation convinced me that I didn't have an acid problem. I had no proof that I ever had an acid problem. I had twenty years of proof that I had a reflux problem.

From the other side of this now, I realize that my doctors' advice wasn't entirely wrong, to address the acid and ensure that I wasn't refluxing massive amounts of acid into my esophagus. Yet it wasn't until I consulted with my more recent doctors (my allergist and current gastroenterologist) that I was assisted in understanding and actually dealing with the core of the problem as the reflux, and not the byproduct effects of the acid.

I also learned, as a small consolation, that most people have some level of reflux, and that the LES isn't necessarily perfect in any of us. Various factors impact the strength of the LES, including how large our meals are, the stress we're under, medications we take, and even the time of day. That's when I started to research how I could strengthen this muscle. (As a previous personal trainer, I was convinced there had to be a way.) Indeed, I learned that there were some options.

Ways to strengthen the LES included avoiding alcohol, caffeine, tight clothing, gas-producing foods, large meals, to lose a few pounds, and to make sure I was drinking enough water. It is also important to select targeted times of the day for exercise when the stomach is empty. In my most startling moment, I came across research that showed that long term use of PPIs (proton pump inhibitors) could actually weaken the LES. I was blown away. (Again, please research this on your own, as I read from so many sources, I can't even recall which one to cite this from.) To then add further insult to injury, I also found out that proton pumps are not just limited to our stomachs. Proton pumps are present in almost all of the cells in our body, including our brain. And PPIs do not just impact the proton pumps in the stomach. I did not go much further down this rabbit hole because I knew it would only produce fear in me. I only knew I had found enough to be ready to make a change.

The pieces all came together to convince me it was time to systematically come off these proton pump inhibitors. I knew I needed to create the best possible environment for my stomach to do what it was created to do, so I started researching the lifestyle changes that would increase the chances of success in going off of the PPIs.

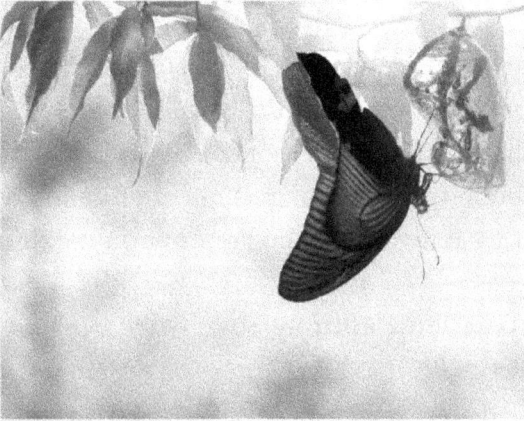

Lifestyle Changes

The first thing I did was to consult my doctor. I now have a wonderful God-fearing gastroenterologist who I trusted with my convictions and my concerns. I told him about my desire to go off the PPIs, and the lifestyle choices I had planned to make. We agreed to do an endoscopy to see where things were, and after the clean results of that, he gave me the green light to go off of them slowly and carefully.

Prior to this endoscopy, which was in February 2022, I had decided to make some radical changes in preparation to go off the meds. These changes are listed on the following pages. I'm not certain I absolutely needed to do all these things, but again, I was determined to create the best possible outcome to go off the PPIs for good. These changes began in late December of 2021, so I had them in place about two months prior to the endoscopy and prior to weaning down the prescription medication.

Gave up caffeine entirely

It took three weeks to stop having headaches, but I made it and realized afterwards that I had the same amount of energy that I had on the caffeine. I was previously drinking three to four cups of regular coffee per day. Later, my friend introduced me to chicory root as a substitute and I fell in love with it! I now drink that and iced herbal tea throughout the day.

Gave up trigger foods

This included alcohol, chocolate, tomatoes, tomato-based sauces, juices, citrus fruits, spicy foods, carbonated drinks including all soda and seltzer, and I cut way back on anything fried. I wasn't sure if these were all going to be permanent changes, but I knew I needed to do them for the time being. I avoided these items strictly for almost a year and then slowly started to introduce a couple of them back into my diet on occasion, and with the right timing and conditions.

Stopped eating late at night

This was as difficult as going off coffee. And sometimes I still find it extremely difficult. I began cutting off all eating after 8:00pm. (I usually go to bed around 11:00pm.) Later in the journey, I moved it to 6:00pm, and now there are occasions where I will eat all my meals by 4:00pm and fast the rest of the day. This alone has made a major difference, and I am certain of that because even when I do all the other things, not doing this will trigger reflux symptoms within the next twenty-four hours. This was a real game-changer for me.

Got a bed wedge and tried to sleep propped up

In my case, this did not work, and started causing me some back problems because I am a side sleeper and couldn't stay on my back. This only lasted for a couple weeks when I realized I couldn't possibly live in a healthy manner if I wasn't sleeping. It probably would be a good change if you are a back sleeper.

I began to drink alkaline water

This was also short-term as I started to get headaches and brain fog after only drinking alkaline water. I know there are a lot of schools of thought on this and the whole topic is somewhat controversial. I am not fully educated on this topic, and it is much more complicated than most people think. I do still occasionally drink it, especially after an acidic meal/drink, but it's a very small percentage of my water intake now. I've heard feedback even from trusted doctors that completely spans the gamut on this, so again, it is best to do your own research.

I started incorporating low-acidic foods

I researched and found foods that I liked that were great for reflux such as:

- Rice
- Pasta
- Bananas
- Oatmeal
- Plantains
- Noodles
- Ginger
- Olive oil
- Watermelon
- Lean meat
- Couscous
- Herbal tea, Chamomile

- Potatoes
- Fish and sushi
- Manuka honey
- Chicory root (my friend introduced me to this as a coffee substitute and it made my journey so much better!)

I began exercising only in the morning

I began a routine to exercise only in the morning, before breakfast, on an empty stomach. Initially this was hard, and I felt very hungry and couldn't wait to eat. I kept the workouts short at that point, usually only ten to fifteen minutes. My body quickly adjusted and now I most enjoy this time of day to workout and am often at the gym for an hour before I go home and enjoy my well-earned breakfast. It's remarkable how God has made our bodies to adapt.

Started incorporating over the counter meds

I did a lot of research to find medications that were the least absorbed by the body, and those with the least side effects, especially long term. For me, that came down to Tagament (Cimetidine 200 mg), Pepcid (Famotidine 20 mg), and Gaviscon Advance. I would take the Pepcid and Tagament a couple times per day with meals, and the Gaviscon Advance thirty minutes after a meal, and at bedtime. After I would take the Gaviscon Advance I would not drink or eat anything for three hours. (I've heard that's about as long as the "seal" lasts, and if you eat/drink before that, you basically break the seal.)

While my allergist initially recommended Gaviscon, my current gastroenterologist helped me to understand that there is a huge difference between the versions made in the US, versus the UK. The US version is aluminum based and my gastroenterologist strongly cautioned against the long-term use of it. The UK version, usually referred to as "Gaviscon Advance" has the active ingredients of sodium alginate & potassium hydrogen carbonate. According to my gastroenterologist, the sodium alginate is the key component here. My understanding is that there are other products with this as the active ingredient, but again, please do your research and also be aware of other ingredients included. My gastroenterologist has currently cleared me for long term use of the UK version of Gaviscon Advance, as needed.

Cut down beverage intake at meals

This is another one that I tried out but don't necessarily subscribe to completely anymore. In some of my research, I found that when we drink a lot with our meals it creates an environment that refluxes easier than if we had just eaten food without a beverage. In theory it makes sense, but I didn't notice a huge difference either way. In fact, it was often more stressful to figure out how to get all my water intake appropriately in, in between meals, without interrupting the efficacy of the "seal" of the Gaviscon. I found that my water intake was more likely to get cut when I was trying to not have a beverage with meals, and then I would get dehydrated, tired, and frustrated altogether.

Began eating smaller meals

This was yet another one that I have adapted a bit. The smaller meals are unquestionably better for digestion and for reflux. I decided to eat four to five smaller meals per day. But it became a lot to coordinate and manage. How do I wait the appropriate time in between meals for the medication to fully work to support the digestion of my last meal without reflux? How do I fit in all those meals and stop eating early in the day? How do I adjust this socially when I'm eating out with friends or family? Should I really now be taking the Gaviscon Advance five to six times per day if I'm taking it with every meal and also at bedtime? It was a lot to handle, and I didn't feel certain I wanted to take that much over-the-counter medication. I also ended up feeling unsatisfied and hungry only eating such small portions and then dreaming of the next time I could eat. For some people who can make this work well, I do recommend it. But for me, it was frustrating, and I knew I needed to minimize the stress of all the changes at once. Instead of many smaller meals, I now typically only eat twice per day. I eat in the morning after working out, and I eat an early dinner. Occasionally, I will have another snack around dinner time with my husband, depending on how many calories I consume. (I manage my weight by regularly counting calories during the week and taking the weekends off.)

I lost a little weight

I didn't have to make much of an effort to lose a little weight. I'm certain that avoiding the tons of coffee creamer that I used to use, cutting back on eating late at night, and cutting out fried foods made a significant difference. I lost between five and ten pounds in the transitional period and felt better in my clothes. It was a positive side effect for sure, finally! Tight clothes are discouraged for those who reflux as it creates more pressure around the stomach and its contents. It was nice to fit more comfortably in my clothes with the weight loss, as I do notice a difference if I'm wearing something that is tighter around my stomach.

Ate lower fat foods

I have also modified this a bit too. While my initial time period to prepare my body for going off the PPIs focused on lower fat foods, I gradually shifted to incorporating more healthy-fat foods. I now also eat fried foods occasionally, but you'll hear more about my present diet in the later part of the book.

Chewed gum after meals

While this is good advice, and sound advice that I had received from my doctor, for me, this was sporadic, and that is only because I wouldn't chew gum once I took the Gaviscon Advance, which was typically thirty-minutes after a meal. It was only when I didn't have access to the Gaviscon Advance that I would chew gum (which does promote digestion and has other benefits as well). When I wasn't eating, I was usually allowing the Gaviscon Advance to work, or fasting at night. There wasn't a lot of time for gum chewing in between although I could do it at night before bedtime, especially if I felt tempted to eat.

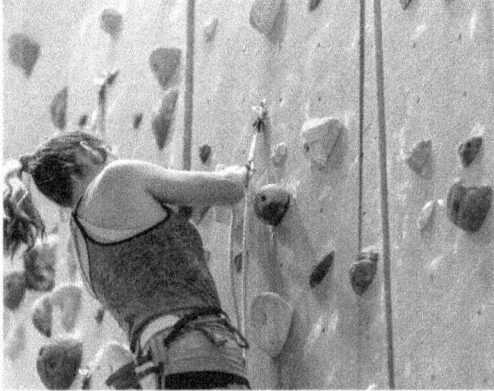

Coming Off Prescription Meds

Immediately after the green light from my gastroenterologist (after my endoscopy) in February 2022, I put together a plan to slowly taper off my prescription PPIs. I knew from experience that going off them slowly was the best way to ensure success.

Earlier in my life, after I had gotten saved (accepted Jesus as my Lord and Savior), I decided then that God was going to heal me of acid reflux and if I prayed and believed it, that it would happen. I prayed, and believed, and went off my prescription medication cold turkey. Several days later, I had some of the worst heartburn of my life, and even though I resisted for a couple of days, I eventually went back on the medication and didn't question it again for a long time.

That was an important lesson for me. While yes, the Bible says that we are to pray and believe that we will receive, we must also understand that our finite minds are incapable of understanding all the ways in which God will answer our prayers. We also must be praying for something that is within His will. When that all comes together, He is faithful to respond. It may not always be the response we are seeking, but there will be a response, and if we are in Christ, the results will always be worked for good (Romans 8:28). In my case, I believe that my prayer at that time was more arrogant than it was reverent. I wasn't praying for my body to be healed because it was His body, His temple. I was praying for my body to be healed so I wouldn't have to deal with the condition anymore. There's a big difference in those two heart postures.

It was pivotal to realize, more than a decade later, that I was put in charge of stewarding something that was not my own but belonged to God. As the manager of this "temple" I needed to not only steward it to the best of my ability, but also to check in with the Owner if there was a problem that I didn't know how to handle. I had to come to the end of myself to say, "God, I am not feeling like this is the way to go, but I want to check with You, because ultimately, this body belongs to You. Whatever You want me to do, I'll do. I just want to care for what is Yours." When I got there, that heart posture changed everything. Then, piece by piece, it all came together for me to walk it out with Him in faith, rather than on my own timing, in self-centered determination.

I printed out a couple of blank monthly calendars and started a medication chart. Beginning on February 2, 2022, I started taking my previously daily PPIs (at the time, I was on Dexilant) every other day. I continued with the lifestyle changes that were mentioned in the previous chapter, including the over-the-counter medications. If there was a day where I was experiencing breakthrough symptoms, I would take an additional Famotidine (Pepcid) or supplement with Tums. I continued taking the Dexilant every other day for three weeks.

Three weeks later, I began my regimen of taking them every third day. I did that for three weeks—also following all the same lifestyle changes throughout this entire process. After those three weeks, I began taking them once per week and I did that for three weeks. On March 31, 2022, I took my last dose of my Dexilant (PPIs) and have not been back on them as of the date of this publication.

For me, this slow tapering worked well. I didn't have many breakthrough symptoms at all. For others, this might not be recommended or might need adjustments. My doctor has given me permission to continue to take the PPIs as needed, but I haven't felt like I've needed them since I've been off them. I am incredibly grateful for what God has done, with the most important work having started in my own heart.

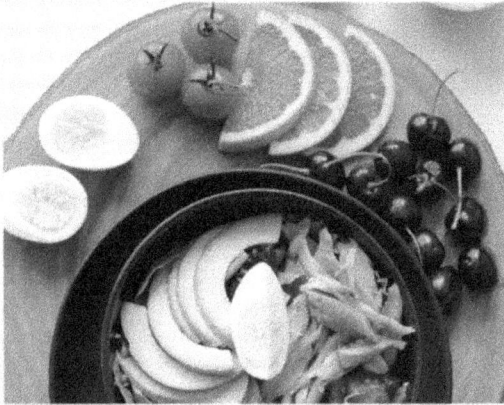

Foods & Supplements

I f you research online for "low acidic" foods, you will find a ton of information. I scoured many of those lists looking for foods that I knew I would be able to enjoy and were sustainable for the lifelong changes that I was needing to make. I knew I couldn't make dietary changes that were going to make me constantly miserable. So aside from the lower acidic foods, I also kept a list of foods that made me feel good after I ate them. It is amazing how much we learn about what we eat if we pay attention to how we feel afterwards. Our bodies will always be honest with us! At the end of this short chapter, I list the foods that I avoided (and mostly still do avoid), and the foods that I ate (included in that list are those that made me feel good also). I would suggest making your own list of foods that make you feel good. The qualifier there is that they make you feel good *after* you eat them—not like typical "comfort foods" that only make us feel good *as* we are eating them. This should not be a mental or emotional thing; this is paying attention to your body and the physical effects of the food you eat to see how your body reacts to it. Remember, God designed our bodies intelligently—not every craving is bad. Sometimes it really is our body trying to communicate what we need.

My so graciously protective husband also wanted to be sure that I had the appropriate supplements to support all the changes I was making. We are both believers that most people don't get enough nutrients out of just food anymore and for that reason, supplementation is wise. One of the most important things I started to add as a supplement was raw aloe (directly from the plant).

Since not every species of aloe plant is edible, it's important to do your research if you go this route. I read a good bit on aloe supplementation and watched many videos until I was convinced that I wanted to try it. I found a store near me that sold edible aloe leaves and I went and brought them home to try them. The taste is awful, truth be told. It is much like what you might imagine eating a bit from a jar of aloe skin protectant would taste like. But I had to admit that it seemed to have positive effects on my stomach, and I couldn't deny all the healing benefits from the proven research on aloe. While I know there are aloe drinks on the market, I am very much an "all or nothing" kind of person, so I figured if I was going with aloe, then I wanted to go with the form that packed the most punch and eating it directly from the plant was that option for me. I typically cut the plant into approximately one-ounce slices, and then I soak them in water for an hour. (I've heard this helps release some of the bitterness from the latex.) I then store the pieces in the refrigerator and eat one piece before each meal. I find the aloe pieces seem to keep well for up to two weeks in the refrigerator. Again, do your research, as aloe can be an allergen for people and is definitely not a solution for everyone. The drinks may also be a more pleasant option as well!

In college, I worked for the retail chain, GNC, which sold vitamins and supplements. I learned a great deal from my time with that company including the fact that most people will take anything as long as the claim on the bottle fits their goal. Please be extremely cautious about supplementing with anything at all. Even vitamins can be toxic if taken in the wrong dosage. It is very important to consult with a qualified physician on how to supplement properly.

These are the current supplements that I take:

- Magnesium Citrate 250mg (x2)
- Iron 65 mg (Vitron C, elemental coated iron)
- Selenium 200 mcg
- Optimized Quercetin 250 mg
- Vit B12 2,500 mcg
- Vit B6 50 mg
- Vit E 180 mg (400 IU)
- Low dose Aspirin 81 mg
- Digestive Advantage Probiotics
- Women's Multivitamin
- Omega-3 100 mg
- Immune Support: Elderberry, Vit C, Vit D, Zinc

These are the foods I avoid:

- Carbonated beverages, including all soda
- Caffeine
- Juice
- Coffee, regular tea
- Chocolate

- Onions
- Anything fried
- Alcohol
- Most processed foods, especially with high-fructose corn syrup
- Citrus
- Tomato-based sauces (although tomato-cream sauces seem to work ok with me)
- Spicy foods
- Anything that I now know doesn't make me feel good! (It's not worth it no matter how I try to convince myself!)

These are the foods I enjoy and incorporate regularly:
(and also make me feel good)

- Manuka honey
- Oatmeal
- Berries
- Watermelon
- Eggs
- Rice
- Sushi
- Bananas
- Plantains
- Noodles

- Ginger
- Olive oil
- Lean meat (all kinds)
- Couscous
- Herbal tea
- Potatoes, especially sweet potatoes
- Bread
- Pasta
- Most cheeses in moderation
- Vitamin Water (XXX Acai Berry is my favorite)
- Spinach
- Naan bread
- Avocado
- Coconut anything
- Rice pudding
- Vanilla wafers
- Lotus Biscoff cookies
- Chicken & dumplins'
- Boba tea
- Oat milk
- Popcorn
- Seafood (all kinds)
- Rice cakes
- Salad (especially with olive or coconut oil)
- Black beans
- Chicken or egg salad

- Natural sugar, most seasonings, and mild spices for food
- Eggplant
- Microgreens (I grow my own)

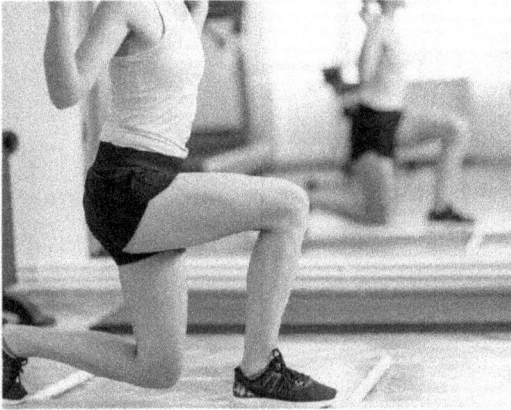

Exercise

As a previous personal trainer, I was alarmed when I heard that exercise could worsen reflux. I knew I was not going to forgo exercise for the rest of my life, and so I began research about what type of exercise would support my healing and not hurt it.

In my research I found that one of the most important aspects of working out with a reflux condition is to do it on an empty stomach whenever possible. Alternately, trying to maintain an upright position will also be more beneficial, especially if you are not working out on an empty stomach.

Typically, since I try not to eat after dinner the night before, I get up in the morning afterwards and do my workout on a completely empty stomach. As I said earlier, this took some getting used to, as I was used to having breakfast before a workout. At first, after those hours of fasting, I didn't feel like I had energy to workout and I wasn't motivated. I just wanted to eat. After a few weeks, my body completely adjusted though, and now I enjoy my morning workouts. Assuming my schedule supports it, I workout up to six days a week, first thing in the morning.

Stretching is the most critical part of my workout time. I typically stretch for about twenty minutes before I start any exercising. I use a foam roller whenever possible as it's the best thing to really work through tight or sore muscles and get them loose again. On the days I don't workout I still try to stretch first thing in the morning.

From my training experience, I've learned that variety is key in getting results from exercise, so I vary my workout every day. There aren't any exercises that I specifically avoid except for anything that would keep me upside down for an extended period of time. (I don't really even know what those would be!) I should also mention that I don't drink water (or anything else) while I'm working out. I realize that might be quite an adjustment for some people, but I've found that leaving my stomach completely empty ensures the best possible conditions to support my workout without triggering reflux.

If I am working out after I have eaten, even if it is several hours, I will avoid anything that has me lying down, or putting a lot of pressure on my stomach. (The pressure on the stomach encourages reflux.) The activities that I avoid in that circumstance includes swimming, pushups, stretching (lying or bending down), and any gym machinery that has me on my stomach (leg crunches) or on my back (stomach, leg, or back machines). If your stomach is full or if you are still digesting, it's best to stay as upright as possible. I also avoid anything that is strenuous in that case, which includes running, even though it is upright. Exercises that I will participate in when my stomach is not empty include walking, light hiking/climbing, light arm weights, light dancing. I have often found that a light walk after a meal helps digestion as well.

Unless a doctor tells you otherwise, don't forgo your workout because you fear reflux. It doesn't make sense to sacrifice a major area of health to try to support another one. There is a way you can do it, you just need to be patient, give yourself some grace to mess it up sometimes, and experiment to find out what exercises support you best. The better you feel, the more sustainable the routine will be. I used to tell my personal training clients to do what they enjoy (in terms of exercise). If you do not enjoy running, you may want to run occasionally to vary your routine, but don't let that be your focus. Don't force yourself to be a runner just because you think it's the best workout. Find a sport or activity you enjoy and you will do it more and with a better attitude as well. You shouldn't be miserable working out. Jesus died to give us abundant life. You have permission to enjoy that within proper stewardship of the blessing of health and holiness.

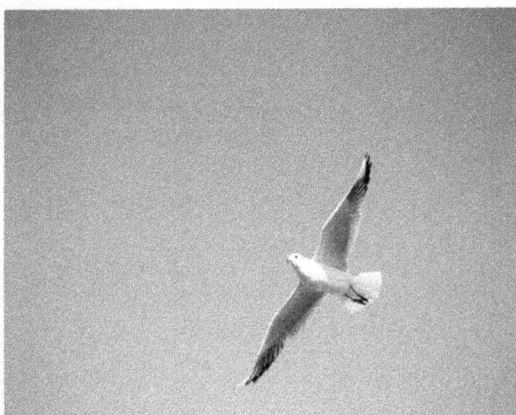

Healing

One year after I went off my PPIs, my gastroenterologist ordered an additional endoscopy just to check the results of the year off the meds. It is with the most heartfelt gratitude and all glory to God that I can say that the results came back clear. I may have an additional endoscopy in three to five years, but I am going to let God make the call on that.

Since the PPIs were the only prescription medications I was taking regularly, I am now completely off prescription medications, and at the age of forty-four, I have never felt better.

My weight is good. I've kept off the ten pounds that I've lost and have since incorporated resistance training into my workouts to keep lean muscle mass. I believe that my overall body fat percentage has decreased even though I don't have a reading of what it was before. I do know now that I am at a "low" body fat percentage for my age and height. I feel good in my clothes, and I don't stress myself out trying to fit into stuff that doesn't fit well or doesn't glorify God.

Thanks to the work of an outstanding dentist and orthodontist, nearly all of the work on my teeth has been completed and I finally have a healthy mouth again. I have spoken to my dentist and confirmed that reflux could have produced or at least greatly influenced a lot of the dental problems I have dealt with. I am not seeing the erosion or effects of the "soft enamel" as I was in the past. I have had clean dental exams for more than a year now. I also must thank my incredibly generous husband for funding all these treatments and more.

My allergies have nearly completely subsided. After almost ten years of regular allergy treatments, I no longer take any allergy medication or shots whatsoever. I do not have any hives at all and am definitely not allergic to my own sweat. (Hallelujah!) I believe I still may have some allergies to certain foods or medications, but I've lived without them for so long, I got used to being without them and have not been through testing again to understand if they are still issues. I'm settled living without the short list of things I avoid. I am amazed that when everyone else is sneezing and coughing through allergy season, I am at ease. Having been on allergy medication since I was a kid, this is a true miracle for me.

In another amazing, unexpected twist, my eyesight has also improved. With each annual eye exam in the past, I have been able to expect that my prescription will be updated and new glasses will need to be purchased. (I wear glasses for distance.) My latest exam, which occurred nearly a year after going off the PPIs, began with the doctor asking me how I felt my vision was, and I told her I believed it had actually improved. Somewhat surprised, she did her exam and confirmed that it had improved. I have never had that happen in all the time that I've been going for regular eye exams, which started in my late teens. She asked me what I was doing differently, and I was happy to share a bit of this story.

I am no longer anemic, and all of my bloodwork came back good at my last exam. I am not deficient in anything. I do continue to take an iron supplement, (since my levels were good while continuing to take it), but I plan to have that rechecked in the future with the hopes that the iron supplement may be unnecessary at some point as well. My blood pressure is that "of a kid" according to the anesthesiologist at my last endoscopy. I am no longer seeing borderline high blood pressure readings.

I have had no lasting LPR symptoms since I went off the PPIs and began this new regiment. If I occasionally eat late, or have a trigger food, or eat a very large meal, I will have some throat clearing, and once in a while, a spontaneous cough or two, but in that case, I will take a Tums, and an additional Famotidine (Pepcid) and then will be sure to always have the Gaviscon Advance before bed. I believe the fasting from late afternoon to morning has also helped my stomach to be used to only consuming a reasonable amount of food. I'm quickly reminded how uncomfortable it is if I push it and eat an extra large meal.

I am still taking the over-the-counter medications as I mentioned earlier, but I've been able to skip a dose of Gaviscon Advance here and there, especially when I am eating lighter. (In that case, I usually can skip the lunch dose.) I do not skip the bedtime dose. At some point, I may also try cutting back on the Tagament or the Pepcid as well to see how that impacts me.

I am sleeping much better. I no longer have any back pain (while I didn't mention it earlier, it was something that seemed to be getting progressively worse with aging as well). I do not cough at night. My breathing is also better, and I sleep much more soundly. I do not have any heartburn symptoms when I lie down or when I wake up.

Finally, I am enjoying my food more than ever. It is amazing how much we take for granted. When I have the occasional chocolate, or small glass of red wine, I savor it slowly and enjoy it to the fullest. If I consume them, I try to enjoy trigger foods earlier in the day, well before bedtime. I am thoughtful about my meals now that I'm usually only eating twice a day. I look forward to what I eat and listen to the cravings of my body within reason and within the boundaries of what I know will generally be beneficial to me. I enjoy healthy fats and do not deprive my body of them. I thank God for the food and ask Him to consecrate it to benefit me (1 Timothy 4:4-5).

I don't feel deprived anymore. (I always believed I would feel this way if I made all of these lifestyle changes! It was a lie!) Instead of going out for coffee, or a drink, I now go to a healthy lunch or breakfast with friends. (And I enjoy my chicory root at home as my own "coffee.") My husband has been wonderfully supportive to join me in "linner" (lunch-dinner) when we go out, and we enjoy less crowded restaurants and our pick of tables when we go around 4:00pm. We also usually get good service at that time as well since the restaurants aren't overloaded.

I still do struggle with not eating late at night (that is still a temptation for sure) but having breached those boundaries enough times to understand the difference in how I sleep and how I feel the next morning, that helps to keep me sustained most of the time. When I get hungry at night, I try to think about what I want to eat and plan for it the next day, so I don't feel like I'm going without it. If this is the biggest cross I have to carry in relation to this issue, I can live with it in gratitude. And most of the time I realize that much of the temptation to eat late at night is based in emotion and comfort even more than hunger. I know that because when I choose to not eat late at night, I don't wake up hungry in the morning, and I sleep better that night.

In relaying my story to a new friend recently, I told her I had been healed from acid reflux and she was confused to find out that I was still taking medicine for it (the over-the-counter medications). She assumed that my "healing" included a complete departure from any treatment or medication.

I know I have been healed of acid reflux because acid was never my main issue. I also believe I have been healed because I now know how to effectively treat the reflux without being on any prescription medication and without being on any medication which has known serious side effects. Despite my incredibly poor choices in the past, God has blessed me with health and has given me a new heart to want to steward my body for His glory. I don't have selfish reasons for taking medication anymore because I am avoiding the more important adjustments I should make. I am now taking a few over the counter medications for proper management alongside responsible decisions.

I can't close this book without mentioning the book my dad intended to write. Once he got sick, he had a massive shift in perspective on life. For the first time, he became dependent on others and the love they could show him. This was quite the shift from the energetic, hard-working, self-driven approach he took to most of his life. He eventually disclosed the humbling revelation that he understood that he would only survive by embracing the love he was being given. He began to write a book which was meant to be his memoir and an inspiration to others. Its title was to be, "Let Yourself Be Loved." My dad passed away on March 31, 2003, exactly nineteen years prior to the date I would officially begin my own healing on this journey.

While my dad didn't complete his book, he did complete his journey. The Lord graciously took him into Heaven and showed him that the answer he had found was indeed correct. Embracing the love that God has set in place for all of us, through His Son, Jesus, is the only way to enduring life. If you haven't done so yet, I invite you to let yourself be loved by the Great Healer.

God didn't have to spare me from the path my relatives traveled, but He did—at least thus far—and I am grateful for the days I've been given and the opportunity to make the lifestyle changes I have. They have all improved my quality of life significantly. I am not suffering. Acid reflux is not something I fear at all anymore. I have indeed been healed, and I am continuing to experience blessings of additional healing still taking place in me. I am believing for even greater results this side of Heaven, and am completely reassured for those on the other side.

All glory and honor to the One who secured it all, and Who alone has healed me, Jesus Christ.

ABOUT THE AUTHOR: JOANNA SANDERS

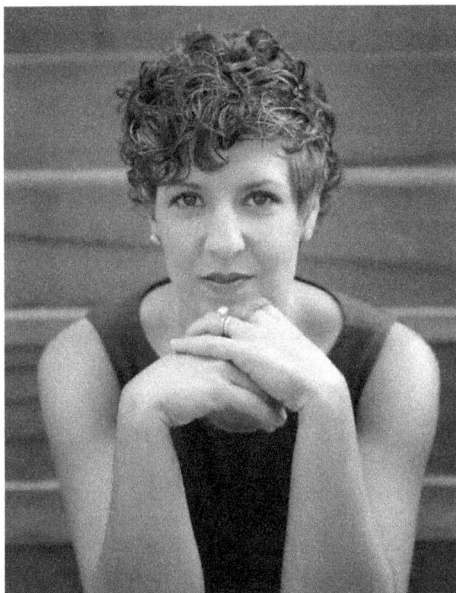

Joanna Sanders is the author of *Fire Women: Sexual Purity & Submission for the Passionate Woman* and the co-author of *DiscipleTrip* with Dr. Joey Cook.

Joanna is a graduate of Villanova University and Moody Theological Seminary. She's the founder and the head writer of Colossians46.com, which provides biblical content support, writing, and editing. Joanna has written for several Christian publications including a weekly blog for *Today's Christian Living* magazine and has a heart for women's ministry.

In 2023, Joanna also became the owner of Triumph Scooter Gear, a Christian centered company that produces apparel for riders and non-riders alike. Joanna's goal with Triumph is to infiltrate the skateparks and the extreme sports community with the light of Christ.

Most importantly, she is wife to Geoff and mom to three godly-men-in-training.

Joanna's books are available on Amazon.com and BarnesandNoble.com.

Connect with Joanna online at www.colossians46.com

Additional copies of this book
may be purchased
on Amazon.com
and BarnesandNoble.com